Y0-CPE-715

## August 1348
The disease appears in London, where King Edward III blames it on a buildup of garbage in the streets.

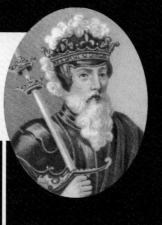

## July 1349
The Black Death reaches the Netherlands, Denmark, Norway, Sweden, Russia, Ireland, and eastern Greenland.

## June 1348
The Black Death reaches England through a port town in Dorset.

## January 1348
The plague reaches Greece, Bulgaria, Russia, Cyprus, and Egypt.

## February 1349
Two thousand Jews are burned alive in Strasburg, Germany, for supposedly creating the plague.

## Spring 1350
The Black Death reaches Scotland, where one-third of the population dies.

**1348**

**1349**

**1350**

## April 1348
People begin to blame Jews for purposely spreading the plague and start attacking European Jewish communities.

## April 1349
Continuing to spread through the British Isles, the plague enters Wales.

## August 1349
The plague enters Poland via a merchant ship from Norway.

## Summer 1348
Religious fanatics called flagellants, who beat themselves in public to persuade God to end the plague, first appear in Germany.

## September 1348
King Edward's daughter contracts the Black Death and soon dies.

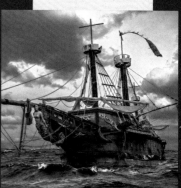

# A Crucial Turning Point in History

"Oh hard death, impious [wicked] death, bitter death," bemoaned Gabriele de Mussis, a prominent lawyer in the Italian city of Piacenza in 1348. These words are part of his riveting written description of the frightening appearance of the so-called Black Death in his community. That disease, which later generations determined to be bubonic plague, spread quickly through Italy and then into other sectors of Europe, always with the same disastrous physical and social effects that de Mussis noted. "Cruel death," he continued,

> divides parents, divorces spouses, parts children, separates brothers and sisters. We bewail our wretched plight [and] the future threatens yet greater dangers. . . . To flee is impossible, to hide futile. Cities, fortresses, fields, woods, highways, and rivers are ringed by . . . evil spirits, the executioners of the supreme Judge [God], preparing endless punishments for us all.[1]

This passage constitutes only a small fraction of de Mussis's scary account of that awful pandemic, which ravaged Europe from autumn 1347 to the early months of 1350. Although in past eras the continent had undergone a number of epidemic diseases, none, before or since, wreaked havoc on the immense scale of the Black Death. Spreading with growing ferocity from town to town and from nation to nation, it devastated entire regions, decimating local populations.

> "Cruel death divides parents, divorces spouses, parts children, separates brothers and sisters."[1]
>
> —Fourteenth-century Italian lawyer Gabriele de Mussis

The exact number of dead will likely never be known, and modern experts differ on the overall death toll. The most conservative estimates say that about 25 million Europeans—roughly a third of the populace at the time—died. Another 50 million people perished in North Africa, the Middle East, and Asia. Other scholars think these figures are far too low. They suggest that the Black Death killed as many as 200 million of the roughly 500 million people then occupying the planet. If true, a staggering 40 percent of the human species then in existence met a gruesome end.

## Europe Forever Changed

Whatever the ultimate death toll was, it accounted for only part of the damage the Black Death did to humanity. The disease caused extreme fear and was often unpredictable, factors that did untold psychological damage. There was no way to know who would be afflicted; the disease struck without regard for gender, age, social position, wealth, or other such factors. On the one hand, it frequently destroyed entire families, neighborhoods, and villages; yet on the other, it was not uncommon for people who were in close contact with plague victims to survive unscathed. Also, no one, including the doctors of the time, knew what caused the plague. Thus, treatments and cures remained elusive.

The combination of all these factors left society overwhelmed with confusion and distress, which insidiously tore asunder the pillars supporting civilized life. The sight and smell of death seemed to be everywhere. In his *Decameron* (ca. 1351), Italy's Giovanni Boccaccio described the "smell of decomposing bodies" in his

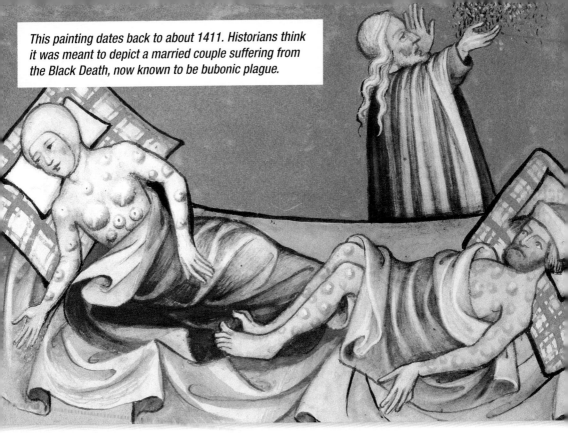

This painting dates back to about 1411. Historians think it was meant to depict a married couple suffering from the Black Death, now known to be bubonic plague.

native city of Florence. "The city was full of corpses. The dead were honored with no tears or candles or funeral mourners; in fact, things had reached such a point that the people who died were cared for as we care for goats today."[2]

The Black Death seemed to largely subside during the 1350s, and over time the bonds holding normal, polite society together were seemingly reestablished. But the ordeal had left Europe forever changed. One major alteration was how large numbers of people now viewed God. Many assumed that he had sent the plague to punish people for their sins, and some began to wonder whether God even existed. As Philip Ziegler, a noted expert on the Black Death, points out, the pandemic created a major crisis of faith: "Assumptions which had been taken for granted for centuries were now in question, [and] the very framework of men's reasoning seemed to be breaking up. . . . The anguish and disruption which [the Black Death] inflicted made the greatest single contribution to the disintegration of an age."[3]

## The Next Destroying Angel

Europe's economic, legal, and educational systems underwent similar large-scale transformations in the disease's wake. These, along with the physical, psychological, and religious tolls, were potent factors in the continent's ongoing transformation from medieval to modern times. Historians therefore see the Black Death's fourteenth-century visitation as a crucial turning point in both European and world history.

Moreover, the historical significance of the bubonic plague was worsened by the fact that the disease did not permanently disappear during the 1350s. Over the ensuing centuries, it repeatedly resurfaced around the globe in small-

> **"The very framework of men's reasoning seemed to be breaking up."[3]**
>
> —Scholar Philip Ziegler

er yet still destructive outbreaks, including in England in 1361 and 1603, France in 1596, Germany in 1632, Denmark in 1710, Turkey in 1801, China in 1894, and the United States in 1900. As these reprises demonstrate, the plague can strike anywhere and at any time, as can outbreaks of other deadly diseases. In the words of popular science writer Richard Conniff, "The one great lesson we should take away from history is this: When [one lethal] pandemic ultimately subsides, we cannot afford to forget [it] happened. We cannot just move on. Somewhere on the planet, the next great pandemic, the next destroying angel, is already taking wing."[4]

# CHAPTER ONE

# The Black Death Assaults Europe

Giovanni Boccaccio and the other fourteenth-century chroniclers of the Black Death were overcome by "horror and disbelief at the number of deaths they saw around them," writes Rosemary Horrox, the foremost modern expert on that medieval pandemic. Singling out the region that was perhaps most devastated by the disease, she points out that "nearly half the population of England died in something like 18 months." Not every European nation suffered that badly, she adds, yet most produced enormous death tolls in the span of a mere two years. "The Black Death," she states, was unarguably "a human disaster of appalling magnitude."[5]

One reason why the bubonic plague managed to kill so many Europeans between 1347 and 1350 was because no one knew what caused it, so there was no cure. Another factor was that no one was prepared for such a massive and lethal onset of disease. For several centuries prior to the Black Death's arrival during the 1300s, disease epidemics had been relatively few—isolated to widely separated regions—and fairly small-scale outbreaks. Among the worst of those ailments was ergotism (then called St. Anthony's fire), caused by a fungus that infests rye and other grains.

Also prevalent in some areas was leprosy, a chronic infection that can badly disfigure the face and limbs. Still, leprosy was not very contagious. And, unlike bubonic plague, it was usually not fatal.

Another reason why the Black Death killed so many Europeans during the fourteenth century was because, at that moment in history, their numbers were larger than they had ever been. Europe's population had grown by more than 300 percent between the late 900s and the early 1300s. By the mid-1300s, therefore, the continent had at least 75 million people, constituting a lot of potential victims. Furthermore, a large proportion of them dwelled in close quarters in cities, which made the spread of any highly infectious disease inevitable. All of these factors contributed to the frighteningly high death toll during the disease's late 1340s assault.

## Where Did It Originate?

Despite the fact that Europeans of that era had no idea what caused the plague and were unprepared for it, they did manage to roughly determine its origins. Numerous writers of that era, including Gabriele de Mussis, reported that the disease came from the "East," the general European designation for the Middle East, India, and central Asia.

Modern historians have verified that hypothesis. Evidence suggests that during the 1200s and early 1300s the disease took hold in north-central Asia in a local population of marmots—small rodents similar to prairie dogs. These creatures interacted with rats, which carried the bacteria to nearby human habitations, and in about 1331 the plague erupted in an unknown number of Chinese villages and towns. According to the late, great American historian William H. McNeill, after at least several million people died, the disease moved westward along the famous trade route known as the Silk Road. That merchant highway consisted of hundreds of *caravanserais,* or trading posts. "What probably happened between 1331 and 1346," McNeill postulated in his classic book *Plagues and Peoples*, was that the Black Death "spread from *caravanserai* to *caravanserai* across Asia and eastern Europe, and moved thence into adjacent human cities wherever they existed."[6]

Supporting this thesis of relentless westward expansion is both archaeological and literary evidence of plague outbreaks along that trade corridor. During the early 1340s, for example, the disease appeared just south of the Silk Road in northern India. During the same period, it passed south of the Caspian Sea and reached into southern Russia, north of the Black Sea, claiming millions of victims along the way.

Among those victims were large numbers of Mongols who were in the midst of conquering large tracts of western Asia. Beginning in the winter of 1345, the invaders moved southward from the vast, grassy steppes lying above the Black Sea into the Crimean peninsula; there, they laid siege to the Genoese colony of Kaffa. (The Genoese, native to the independent Italian nation of Genoa, were active traders who established colonies along the Black Sea coasts.)

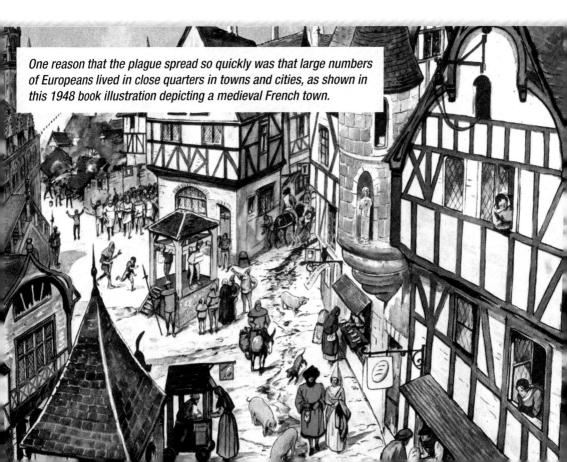

One reason that the plague spread so quickly was that large numbers of Europeans lived in close quarters in towns and cities, as shown in this 1948 book illustration depicting a medieval French town.

The Mongol besiegers decided to take advantage of the fact that the plague was killing many in their ranks by using the victims' corpses as weapons. According to de Mussis, the Mongol commander ordered the bodies

> to be placed in catapults and lobbed into the city in the hope that the intolerable stench would kill everyone inside. What seemed like mountains of dead were thrown into the city, and the Christians could not hide or flee or escape from them. . . . One infected man could carry the poison to others, and infect people and places with the disease by look alone. No one knew, or could discover, a means of defense.[7]

## Bacterial Journeys

Finally convinced that Kaffa would shortly fall to the invaders, a number of the Genoese boarded what ships they still had and sped southward. Eventually they reached the Aegean Sea and then the greater Mediterranean Sea beyond. The escapees had no inkling that an invisible cargo of death lurked in their vessels' holds.

Indeed, beneath the humans' feet, three lesser species were already interacting in a lethal biological progression. The tiniest of the three were the plague germs, which were members of a species of bacteria now called *Yersinia pestis.* Those microbes flourished in the blood of infected rats, which constituted the second species. The third species consisted of fleas that dwelled in the rodents' fur. When the fleas bit the rats to feast on their blood, they consumed the germs infesting that fluid. Some of the infected insects later jumped onto either other rats or human hosts, and when the fleas bit those hosts, the disease's treacherous journey from rat blood to human bodies was complete.

The second crucial journey the plague bacteria undertook happened within the human host and helped to account for the pandemic's enormous death toll. Having made it into the human bloodstream, the microscopic invaders swiftly moved to the lymph nodes in the underarms and lower abdomen. There, they rapidly formed colonies that grew into egg-shaped lumps that came to be known as *buboes*. Calling them "early ornaments of black death," Ieuan Gethin, a popular Welsh poet, vividly described those black sores, which he saw firsthand in 1349:

> Woe is me of the shilling in the arm-pit; it is seething, terrible, wherever it may come, a head that gives pain and causes a loud cry, a burden carried under the arms, a painful angry knob [that] is of the form of an apple, like the head of an onion, a small boil that spares no-one. Great is its seething, like a burning cinder, a grievous thing of an ashy color. It is an ugly eruption that comes with unseemly haste.[8]

Not long after the buboes appeared, some victims saw those sores begin to shrink, and they slowly recovered. But for at least a third of those infected, the bacteria's second journey continued with a vengeance; the germs then attacked the vital organs, in particular the lungs and spleen. At that point, recovery was no longer a realistic option. The victims began bleeding from the anus and/or the skin, and death fairly quickly ensued.

## Like an Unstoppable Tsunami

Some of these alarming symptoms were already apparent among several of the passengers of the Genoese ships that passed from the Black Sea into the Aegean and Mediterranean in 1346 and 1347. Along the way, most of those vessels stopped briefly in Constantinople, the great port city situated on the Black Sea's southern rim. There, rats scurried from boat to boat, transfer-

# A Third of the Human Race Killed?

As the plague headed westward through Europe, it reached England and eventually Scotland. There, a local writer, John of Fordun, penned a tract describing the disease's onslaught in 1350:

> There was a great pestilence and mortality of men in the kingdom of Scotland, and this pestilence also raged for many years before and after in various parts of the world. So great a plague has never been heard of from the beginning of the world to the present day, or been recorded in books. For this plague vented its spite so thoroughly that fully a third of the human race was killed. At God's command, moreover, the damage was done by an extraordinary and novel form of death. Those who fell sick of a kind of gross swelling of the flesh lasted for barely two days. This sickness befell people everywhere, but especially the middling and lower classes. . . . It generated such horror that children did not dare to visit their dying parents, nor parents their children, but fled for fear of contagion as if from leprosy or a serpent.

Quoted in Martha Carlin, "The Black Death in the British Isles," Department of History, University of Wisconsin–Milwaukee. https://sites.uwm.edu/carlin.

ring the plague germs to hundreds of ships bound for Syria, Egypt, Libya, Greece, Italy, France, and Spain. Reacting to the subsequent outbreaks in those places, a Byzantine chronicler remarked, "A plague attacked almost all the seacoasts of the world and killed most of the people."[9]

That writer did not exaggerate by much. The death rate from the disease in the Mediterranean's coastal regions was usually at least 30 percent and soared much higher in some areas. This incredible degree of lethality caught the eye of Baldassarre Buonaiuti, a contemporary businessman and historian native to Florence. When the disease "caught hold in a household," he wrote, "it often happened that not a single person escaped death. And it wasn't just men and women. Even sentient animals such as dogs and cats, hens, oxen, donkeys, and sheep, died from that same disease and . . . almost none who displayed those symptoms, or very few indeed, effected a recovery."[10]

From Europe's Mediterranean ports, the plague proceeded to creep inland like a slow-moving but unstoppable tsunami. French monk and author Jean de Venette witnessed and described the devastation of southern and central France, saying that nothing like it had ever been seen before. In many areas, he stated, "not

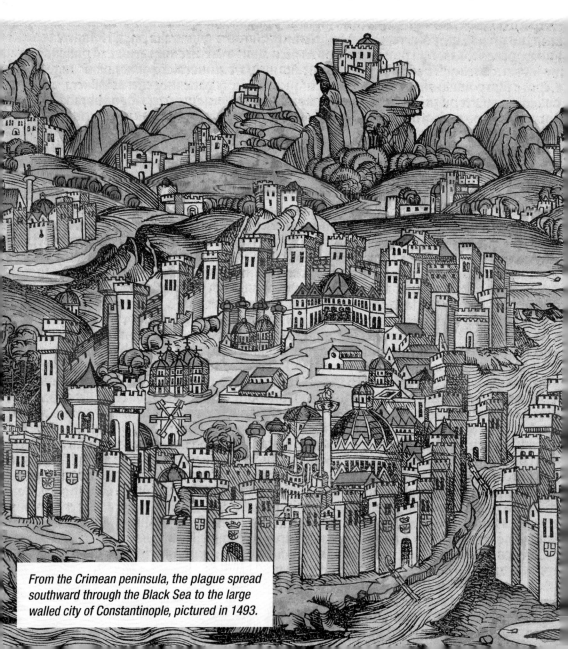

*From the Crimean peninsula, the plague spread southward through the Black Sea to the large walled city of Constantinople, pictured in 1493.*

two men remained alive out of twenty. The mortality was so great that, for a considerable period, more than 500 bodies a day were being taken in carts from the Hotel-Dieu in Paris for burial in the cemetery of the Holy Innocents."[11]

Northern France suffered similarly, after which the wave of misery and death reached across the English Channel to England. English leaders had hoped that the wide waterway would be a barrier to the plague's onslaught. But this hope was dashed in the last months of 1348, when the disease plowed into the southern regions of the British Isles. There, Geoffrey le Baker, a chronicler based in Oxford, summed up the resulting ruin, saying, "This great pestilence, which began at [the port of] Bristol on 15th August and in London about 29th September, raged for a whole year in England so terribly that it cleared many country villages entirely of every human being."[12] Subsequently, some of those who fled in terror from southern and central England unwittingly carried the plague into adjoining regions. By the end of 1349, therefore, the disease had reached northward into the Scottish highlands and across the Irish Sea to Ireland.

## A Deadly Noose Around Europe

Meanwhile, some of the merchants and other travelers who had carried the plague northward through France also headed eastward into Germany. After decimating numerous German villages and cities, the disease continued its death march toward the east, reaching Moscow. There, it killed a powerful grand duke as well as the influential patriarch of the Russian Orthodox Church, along with several million lesser-known individuals.

That high-born individuals and low-born peasants both died in huge numbers is not surprising, as the *Yersinia pestis* microbes did not favor poor people over those with wealth and high status. The Black Death brought low wealthy and poor people alike, as Florence's Buonaiuti noted. Numerous wealthy men and women, he reported, "were borne from their house to church in their coffin with just four undertakers and a lowly cleric carrying the cross."

As in most aspects of life, people of lesser means were given little dignity in death. Most were thrown into cramped spaces in the large mass graves dug by the thousands throughout the continent. Near every church, Buonaiuti went on,

> pits were dug, down to the water-table, as wide and deep as the parish was populous; and therein, whosoever was not very rich, having died during the night, would be shouldered by those whose duty it was, and would either be thrown into this pit, or they would pay big money for somebody else to do it for them. The next morning there would be very many in the pit. Earth would be taken and thrown down on them; and then others would come on top of them, and then earth on top again, in layers, with very little earth, like garnishing lasagna with cheese. The gravediggers who carried out these functions were so handsomely paid that many became rich.[13]

After assaulting Moscow, the Black Death headed southward and struck the Russian cities of Kiev and Odessa, lying directly north of the Black Sea. A number of Russians and other Europeans noted that the deadly plague had taken a long, meandering, tortuous route to reach that area. It had moved westward from Asia into the Crimea; then southward through the Black, Aegean, and Mediterranean Seas to Europe's southern coasts; northward through France and Britain; and then eastward into Germany and Russia. In the words of the late historian David Herlihy, "Launched at Kaffa in the Crimea, and now attaining Kiev," the disease had "closed a deadly noose around Europe."[14]

## A Breakdown of Society's Rules

Many thousands of people died each day inside that immense geographical lasso, and it became widely common to view the slaughter as seemingly unending. De Mussis, Boccaccio, de Venette, and other writers of that era frequently pointed out the failings of doctors and other healers in making headway against the disease. In fact, physicians often contracted it themselves and became lost among the piles of corpses in the ever-present mass graves.

In the meantime, social norms and law and order repeatedly receded before the plague's ceaseless onslaught. In Florence, for instance, Boccaccio described how ordinary respect for both religious and governmental rules

> "Large numbers of men and women abandoned their city, their homes, their relatives, their estates, and their belongings."[15]
>
> —Fourteenth-century Florentine writer Giovanni Boccaccio

had broken down and been extinguished in our city. For like everybody else, those ministers and executors of the laws who were not either dead or ill were left with so few subordinates that they were unable to discharge any of their duties. Hence everyone was free to behave as he pleased. . . . Some people, pursuing what was possibly the safer alternative, callously maintained that there was no better or more efficacious [effective] remedy against a plague than to run away from it. Swayed by this argument, and sparing no thought for anyone but themselves, large numbers of men and women abandoned their city, their homes, their relatives, their estates, and their belongings and headed for the countryside.[15]

Even within families, the normal social order frequently disintegrated. Boccaccio famously reported that siblings abandoned each other and their parents, parents abandoned their children,

When the Black Death swept out of Asia during the mid-1300s, it struck not only Europe but also northern Africa, where most areas were then controlled by Muslim rulers. Some of the major devastation in the region was reported by an eyewitness, noted Arab scholar Ibn Khaldun, who said, in part, that a terrible disease overwhelmed entire countries and wiped out many local populations. It also demolished a number of local ruling families, greatly reducing their power and influence, and some of those families completely disappeared. He added,

> Civilization decreased with the decrease of mankind. Cities and buildings were laid waste, roads and way signs were obliterated, settlements and mansions became empty, dynasties and tribes grew weak. The entire inhabited world changed. The East, it seems, was similarly visited. . . . It was as if the voice of existence in the world had called out for oblivion and restriction, and the world responded to its call. God inherits the earth and whomever is upon it.

Quoted in Michael Dols, *The Black Death in the Middle East.* Princeton, NJ: Princeton University Press, 1977, p. 67.

and husbands deserted wives (or vice versa). Similarly, families abandoned their pets and farm animals. Tragically, a number of plague victims who might have survived the disease ended up starving to death because they were abandoned.

## The Awful March of Death

Hence, Boccaccio went on, "since they had no one to assist them or attend to their needs, they inevitably perished almost without exception. Many dropped dead in the open streets." Others, he said, "though dying in their own houses, drew their neighbors' attention more by the smell of their rotting corpses." Moreover, due to this overall lack of assistance for the gravely ill, "the number of dead soared to incredible heights." The death toll in Florence, Boccaccio declared, "was so enormous that it astonished all who heard tell of it, to say nothing of the people who actually witnessed the carnage."[16]

The specific death toll in Florence, to which Boccaccio referred, is still not known. Most modern scholars, however, speculate that sixty thousand Florentines—constituting about half the city's population—perished between 1347 and 1349. It is likely, furthermore, that around 80 percent of those fatalities occurred in 1348 alone.

Other local European death tolls were similar. Siena, located roughly 40 miles (64 km) south of Florence, lost upward of seventy thousand citizens. Meanwhile, some 130 miles (209 km) to the northeast, in Venice, the Black Death claimed at least one hundred thousand people. Other European cities and nations suffered no less. In France, Paris lost a minimum of fifty thousand people; in England, London had more than one hundred thousand plague victims; and in Germany, where some 170,000 villages had existed before the 1340s, by the early 1400s all but 40,000 of them had been completely depopulated and abandoned.

Overall, the stench of death and the fear of becoming still another doomed victim left a majority of Europeans in a very real sense both terrified and shell-shocked. De Mussis summed up the general feelings of dread and despair that gripped the continent in those few short but calamitous years. "The terrible violence of death running through the world [and] threatening ruin," he wrote, "devoured mortals by a sudden blow. Mourn, mourn you peoples, and call upon the mercy of God."[17]

# CHAPTER TWO

# Trying to Explain the Unexplainable

"In the month of August, 1348, after Vespers when the sun was beginning to set," Frenchman Jean de Venette reported,

a big and very bright star appeared above Paris, toward the west. It did not seem, as stars usually do, to be very high above our hemisphere but rather very near. [Later] . . . when night had come, this big star, to the amazement of all of us who were watching, broke into many different rays and, as it shed these rays over Paris toward the east, totally disappeared and was completely annihilated.[18]

De Venette was one of a number of educated Europeans who suggested that this conspicuous heavenly display might be an omen, or foreshadowing of future events. In particular, he said that it might be a cause of "the amazing pestilence to come, which, in fact, followed very shortly in Paris and throughout France and elsewhere."[19] The disease of which he spoke, of course, was none other than the bubonic plague, or Black Death.

In reading de Venette's chronicle today, scientists are fairly sure that the bright object that broke up in the atmosphere above Paris in 1348 was a meteor, not an omen or cause of the plague. What makes that account stand out so much now is that it was one of many theories proposed by fourteenth-century Europeans to explain why a deadly disease was killing millions of their number. Several of the other proposed explanations were no less misguided. For example, during the mid-1340s tales floated into Europe describing huge storms. Supposedly, they had ravaged India, China, and other Far Eastern lands that were still largely mysterious to most Europeans. Some learned individuals in Italy, France, and neighboring nations wondered aloud whether those distant tempests might somehow have carried the disease into Europe.

Another natural phenomenon cited as a cause of the Black Death during its massive assault on Europe was a supposed series of large earthquakes. Most of them, like the giant storms, were based mainly on rumor and were not documented. But fear of the plague was so rampant that people—educated and uneducated alike—grasped at any explanation that seemed even remotely believable. Thus, it was hypothesized that the earthquakes had unleashed some unknown or unseen poison that made people deathly ill.

## Corrupted Air and Other Natural Explanations

The root cause of most of this unfounded conjecture was the fact that no one in medieval times knew about the existence of germs. Therefore, they had no clue that bacteria—invisible to the naked eye—caused the plague. Hence, all sorts of ideas—some seemingly logical and others far less so—were cited to explain the continent-wide catastrophe. In addition to earthquakes, storms, and falling stars, other baseless entries in the natural phenomenon category included heavy blankets of fog that appeared in parts of Europe in 1347 and supposed realignments of the planets Jupiter, Mars, Venus, and Saturn.

By far the most frequent speculation among the explanations that featured odd happenings in nature was the notion that the air people breathed on a daily basis had somehow become unclean, corrupted, or tainted. Numerous educated people of the day, among them large numbers of doctors, some astronomers, and plenty of literary scholars, readily accepted this theory. In October 1348, several French physicians assembled, discussed the crisis, and issued a joint statement that stated, in part, that the disease could sometimes be caused by the corruption of water or food, as seen in large-scale famines. Yet, they asserted,

we still regard illnesses proceeding from the corruption of the air as much more dangerous. This is because bad air is more noxious than [bad] food or drink in that it can penetrate quickly to the heart and lungs to do its damage. We believe that the present epidemic or plague has arisen from air corrupt in its substance, and not changed in its attributes. By which we wish it [to] be understood that air, being pure and clear by nature, can only become putrid or corrupt by being mixed with something else, that is to say, with evil vapors. What happened was that the many vapors . . . mixed with the air and spread abroad by frequent gusts of wind.[20]

These doctors suggested a number of different possible ways that the air could have been rendered so dangerous to human and animal life. All agreed that one way the air could become poison-ous was to mingle with fumes rising from rotting matter, including the carcasses of dead people and animals. The huge numbers of decaying bodies in slaughterhouses were frequently cited in this regard. To solve this problem, some author-ities proposed cleaning up the streets and slaughterhouses. Rosemary Horrox points out that another common recommenda-tion was "to surround oneself with pleasant smells. No one could avoid breathing, and therefore it was sensible to try to create a barrier of aromatic vapors through which the bad air could not penetrate. This could be achieved indoors by burning spices or wood, such as juniper, which produce aro-matic smoke."[21]

> "We believe that the pres-ent epidemic or plague has arisen from air corrupt in its substance."[20]
>
> —From a 1348 statement by a panel of French doctors

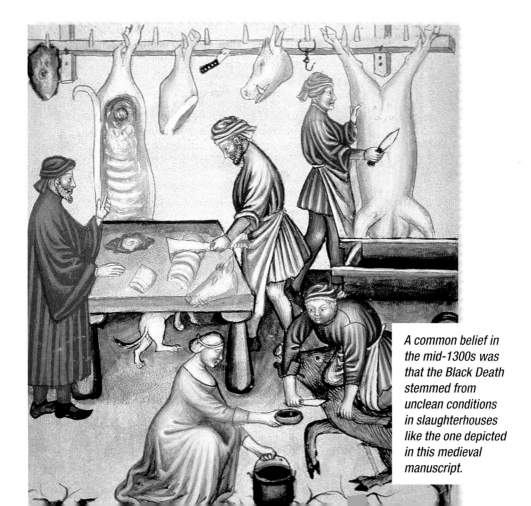

A common belief in the mid-1300s was that the Black Death stemmed from unclean conditions in slaughterhouses like the one depicted in this medieval manuscript.

## Blaming Society's So-Called Undesirables

Corrupted air turned out to be one of the three most widely accepted explanations for the plague's 1340s visitation. Considerably more common, as well as more mean-spirited and dangerous, was the belief that certain undesirable members of society were purposely causing the widespread death and misery. Typically, these people lived outside of society's mainstream and, even in normal times, were seen as uncouth or suspicious.

People who were mentally ill and physically challenged, for example, were frequently suspected of being malicious or somehow touched by evil spirits. Also, if they were very old and unkempt, or lived on society's fringes, some people worried they might be witches. "On the edges of many villages, in poor huts made of sticks and straw, lived outcasts of various kinds," historian James C. Giblin writes. He continues,

> Some were deformed from birth, others were simple-minded, still others were insane. The villagers gave them names like Poor Tom and Mad Mag. The majority were harmless, although children sometimes taunted them and called the old women witches. Most adults simply left them alone. That changed when the Black Death came. . . . Maybe the children were right, [many villagers] thought. Maybe Mad Mag really was a witch. If they got rid of her, maybe the pestilence would finally go away.[22]

Another category of people frequently blamed for causing the plague, or at least making it worse, were heretics. In the words of Shaina Lucas, an expert on the medieval period,

> The definition of a heretic is one who rejects doctrines from the church and their faith. Most examples are a person who was baptized in a certain faith and then rejects that faith. Witches can technically be considered heretics

since most Wiccans and pagans are born and baptized in a different faith from Christianity or Judaism. . . . Heretics were blamed for the Black Death for the reasons of God punishing them for rejecting their original faith.[23]

## The Jews and Extreme Anti-Semitism

Equally misguided and unfair was the common belief that Jews had somehow engineered the plague in a nefarious effort to exterminate Christians. Supposedly, Jews had secretly used disease-ridden powders to poison wells and other water sources. Anxious Christians "now refuse to drink water from wells," a musician working for a high-placed Italian churchman wrote in April 1348. As a result, numerous Jews "were burned for this and are being burned daily, for it was ordered that they be punished thus."[24]

## Planetary Influences

One of the many theories bandied about during the 1300s to explain the assault of the Black Death was that various planetary influences had created it. According to the renowned modern expert on that medieval pandemic, Rosemary Horrox,

> Belief in the influence of the planets was central to medieval science. The universe was seen as an integrated system in which, as in the human body, the condition of one part had a bearing on the health of the others. The earth stood at its center, with seven planets circling it: the moon, Mercury, Venus, the sun, Mars, Jupiter and Saturn. . . . [Regarding the plague,] astrologers argued that Jupiter drew up vapors, which were themselves hot and wet and therefore had an affinity with that planet from the earth. The vapors were then ignited by Mars, an exceedingly hot, dry planet, and in burning produced poisonous fumes. These fumes were blown about the world by the strong southerly winds generated by Jupiter, killing men, animals, and plants. . . . [Many] doctors felt that the action of corrupt [planetary vapors] on the humors [bodily fluids] provided an adequate explanation of all aspects of the plague.

Rosemary Horrox, trans. and ed., *The Black Death*. Manchester, UK: Manchester University Press, 1994, pp. 102–6.

Jews had long been blamed for all sorts of social ills and crimes, so the idea that they were responsible for the Black Death was also widely accepted. Anti-Semitism had existed in Europe for centuries, and it reached a horrifying and brutal peak with the onset of the plague. To his credit, the reigning pope, Clement VI, issued a decree calling upon Christians to refrain from violence against Jews. But few Christians obeyed that edict. Enormous numbers of Jews were defamed, attacked, robbed, and massacred by angry mobs between 1348 and 1350. According to a document penned by a German churchman of that time, all the Jews in the German town of Horw were tossed into a large pit containing wood and straw and burned. When that kindling had been consumed, the churchman wrote, "some Jews, both young and old, still remained half alive. The stronger of [the Christians] snatched up [clubs] and stones and dashed out the brains of those trying to creep out of the fire."[25]

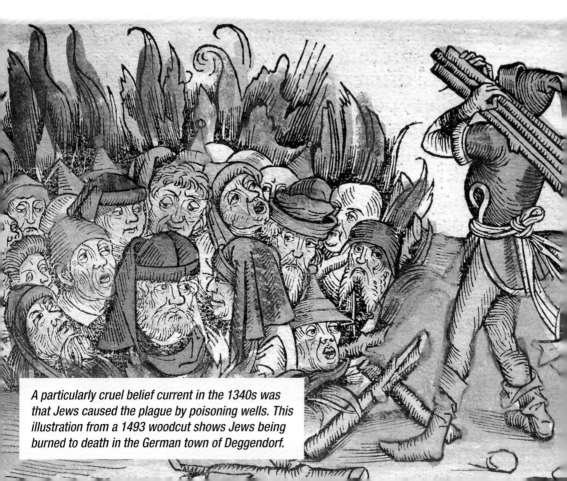

A particularly cruel belief current in the 1340s was that Jews caused the plague by poisoning wells. This illustration from a 1493 woodcut shows Jews being burned to death in the German town of Deggendorf.

Some Jews did confess to poisoning water sources after they were fiendishly tortured by local authorities. A surviving medieval document records how Swiss officials tortured a Jewish man so relentlessly that he finally admitted to the charges against him. The confession he was forced to sign said, in part, "[I] prepared [some] poison and venom in a thin, sewed leather-bag. [I planned to] distribute it among the wells, cisterns, and springs about Venice and the other places to which you [Christians] go, in order to poison [you]."[26]

Even though the accusation was false and the confession made under duress, it and other similar admissions gave Christian authorities throughout Europe what they viewed as a suitable excuse to murder Jews. Modern historians estimate that during the late 1340s at least sixty large European Jewish communities were annihilated as punishment for unfounded accusations of spreading the plague. Moreover, more than a hundred smaller Jewish communities were eradicated as well—and for the same reason.

## The Wrath of the Deity

Although corrupted air and Jewish conspiracies were topics of widespread speculation and discussion during those plague years, by far the most common explanation for the crisis was that it was a manifestation of God's wrath. An English churchman, the prior of Christchurch, ably summed up this argument in September 1348, declaring that God oversaw both the earth and human civilization and that the sins he had witnessed in recent times had angered him. Thus, the Almighty had decided to bring down the Black Death upon humanity as a punishment. "Those whom he loves he censures and chastises," the prior wrote. "That is, he punishes their shameful deeds in various ways during this mortal life so that they might not be condemned eternally. He often allows plagues, miserable famines, conflicts, wars, and

> "[God] often allows plagues . . . to arise, and uses them to terrify and torment men and so drive out their sins."[27]
>
> —Written by an English clergyman in 1348

## Suspicions the Plague Might Be Infectious

From simple observations of the plague's effects on human and animal victims, some inhabitants of medieval Europe came to suspect that the disease might be infectious in some unknown way. Therefore, some people were cautious and tried to avoid close contact with victims of the Black Death. A number of fourteenth-century documents confirm this trend, including a letter penned by French musician Louis Heyligen, who said, in part,

> Because of the growing strength of this disease it has come to pass that, for fear of infection, no doctor will visit the sick (not if he were to be given everything the sick man owns), nor will the father visit the son, the mother the daughter, the brother the brother, the son the father, the friend the friend, the acquaintance the acquaintance, not any blood relation, unless, that is, they wished to die suddenly along with them. . . . For fear of death, men do not speak with anyone whose kinsman or kinswoman has died, because it has often been observed that when one member of a family dies, almost all the rest follow.

Quoted in Catalin Negru, "*History of the Apocalypse:* The Black Plague and the Flagellants," Reason and Religion, 2020. https://reasonandreligion.org.

other forms of suffering to arise, and uses them to terrify and torment men and so drive out their sins."[27]

A fellow Englishman, Thomas Brinton, the bishop of Rochester, later echoed that thought, saying, "We are not stable in faith. We are not honorable in the eyes of the world. On the contrary we are . . . false and in consequence are not loved by God."[28] An anonymous third Englishman of the period cried out, "See how England mourns, drenched in tears. The people stained by sin, quake with grief. Plague is killing men and beasts. Why? Because vices rule unchallenged here."[29] Meanwhile, in distant Italy, Boccaccio more concisely called the onset of the plague "God's just wrath as a punishment to mortals for our wicked deeds."[30]

The God of Abraham, whom Christians, Jews, and Muslims worship, was not the only deity people blamed for unleashing the

Black Death. According to the late, award-winning scholar of the medieval era Barbara W. Tuchman, "Scandinavians believed that a Pest Maiden emerged from the mouth of the dead in the form of a blue flame and flew through the air to infect the next house. In Lithuania, the Maiden was said to wave a red scarf through the door or window to let in the pest."[31]

## Contagious in Some Manner?

Fourteenth-century Europeans resorted to virtually all of these explanations for the plague's assault—from storms and earth-quakes to corrupted air and divine punishment—out of scientific ignorance. They simply knew nothing of the existence of germs. Therefore, they did not conceive of the concept of microscopic infection.

Nevertheless, a number of people of that time did observe features and details of the disease that suggested that it was contagious—that it could somehow pass from person to person. They just had no idea *how.* Boccaccio was among a number of influential public figures who speculated that the plague might be contagious. In his renowned *Decameron,* he observed,

> Touching bread or any other object which had been han-dled or worn by the sick would transport the sickness from the victim to the one touching the object. . . . The pesti-lence I have been describing was so contagious, that not only did it visibly pass from one person to another, but also, whenever an animal other than a human being touched anything belonging to a person who had died from the disease, I say not only did it become contaminated by the sickness, but also died [from it].[32]

The Sicilian Franciscan friar and chronicler Michele da Piaz-za agreed and proposed a specific and, for the time, insightful cause for the plague. "Breath spread the infection among those speaking together," he asserted, "with one infecting the other, and it seemed as if the victim was struck all at once by the affliction and was, so to speak, shattered by it."[33]

Moreover, da Piazza stated, often many ordinary, largely uneducated people seemed to sense the disease's infectious feature. His narrative describing the plague's attack on Messina, in Sicily, points out that the locals frequently sought to avoid contact with victims and perceived carriers of the plague:

> The people of Messina, realizing that the death racing through them was linked with the arrival of the Genoese galleys, expelled the Genoese from the city and harbor with all speed. But the illness remained in the city and subsequently caused enormous mortality. It bred such loathing that if a son fell ill of the disease, his father flatly refused to stay with him, or, if he did dare to come near him, was infected in turn and was sure to die himself after three days. Not just one person in a house died, but the whole household, down to the cats and the livestock, followed their master to death."[34]

In fact, in a world in which both the cause of and remedy for the Black Death remained unknown, death was one of only two certain aspects of the disease. The other was that no one, regardless of social station, was immune. The grave inscription for a prominent churchman of the time, Cardinal La Grange, made the point that both the great and humble were susceptible to the disease, "whatever their condition, age, or sex." And, as the inscription noted, all who succumbed to the plague could expect the same outcome: "dust you are and unto dust you shall return, rotten corpse, morsel and meat for worms."[35]

# Attempts to Deal with the Plague

Although no one in fourteenth-century Europe—or other parts of the world, for that matter—knew what caused the Black Death, they vigorously sought to avoid it and stop its spread. The nature of these overt reactions to the disease varied widely. In Florence, for instance, Boccaccio observed that some citizens "thought moderate living and the avoidance of excess had a great deal to do with avoiding illness, so they lived apart from others in small groups. They congregated and shut themselves up in houses where no one had been sick . . . trying their best not to speak of or hear any news about the death and illness outside."[36]

In contrast to those who closed themselves off from their neighbors, Boccaccio wrote that there were people "of the opposite opinion." These individuals, he wrote, felt that indulging themselves in lighthearted activities was a better way to keep from contracting the disease:

> They believed that drinking a good deal, enjoying themselves, going about singing and having fun, satisfying all their appetites as much as they could, laughing and joking was sure medicine for any illness. Thus, doing exactly as they prescribed, they spent

day and night moving from one tavern to the next, drinking without mode or measure, or doing the same thing
in other people's homes, engaging only in those activities
that gave them pleasure.[37]

These are only two of many general reactions to the plague
by ordinary people. There were also diverse approaches taken
by doctors of that era, many of whom regularly advocated ineffective medical treatments for the disease. Their efforts proved to
be a hit-and-miss process filled with guesswork because, after
all, the medical establishment did not yet know what caused the
Black Death. Nevertheless, a few doctors, along with some logical and enterprising local town officials, gave advice or instituted
public regulations that did sometimes prove effective against the
contagion.

## Relying on Doctors of the Past

Most fourteenth-century European doctors employed ineffective
remedies for the plague. Often, this was because they followed the
disease treatments that had been established by physicians of the
past. In particular, medieval medical practitioners utilized the theories and methods of the ancient Greco-Roman doctor Galen. He
was an extremely important figure during his own era—the second
century CE—and during the dozen centuries that followed.

In large part this was because Galen was one of the smartest,
most thorough, and most inventive medical researchers in human
history. Some of the ideas and techniques he developed were
revolutionary for their time and largely scientifically correct. He
was one of the first doctors in history, for instance, to thoroughly
dissect animals to learn how their organs worked. He was also
the first person to recognize the difference between arterial blood
(blood flowing away from the heart) and venous blood (blood
flowing from the organs back into the heart.)

Despite his brilliance and many accomplishments, however,
many of Galen's theories were incorrect. He did not know about

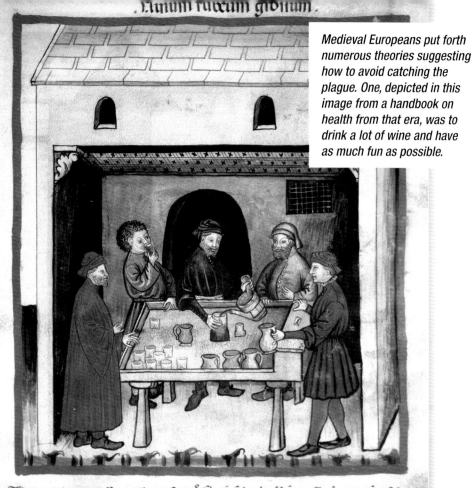

Medieval Europeans put forth numerous theories suggesting how to avoid catching the plague. One, depicted in this image from a handbook on health from that era, was to drink a lot of wine and have as much fun as possible.

Uinum rubeum groſſim. ɔpɫo. ca.ꝛ ſic. in². Electo ſplendioꝛū bn̄ trauſfluecs. uiuamitꝰ ſoꝺaꞇ ſincoptin. nocumtun p̄ſtaꞇ epatiꝛſpleni ꝺebiliḃꝛ. Remō nocumiꞇi cū grani̇anꝰ acetoſis. Qꝺ gnā—ꞇ colām rubeā ɔuenic mag. friꝯ ꝺecrepitis. bꝛeme ꞇ.friꝯ regiomḃꝛ .

germs, of course. Especially crucial, moreover, was the fact that in Rome, where he practiced, it was illegal to dissect human bodies. As a result, some of his conclusions about human anatomy were wrong. The problem was that European doctors in later centuries came to believe that he was an infallible genius whose writings remained the last word in all medical matters. Hence, fourteenth-century physicians did little or no research of their own and instead blindly accepted what Galen had said long before.

Among Galen's incorrect medical concepts were his conclusions about the causes of sickness and disease. He advocated, for example, that those causes included eating or drinking too much; the temperature of the air people breathe; and human personality traits, such as laziness or being too emotional. Following these supposedly correct precepts, when the bubonic plague struck Europe during the 1300s, physicians often advised their patients that they could avoid contracting the disease by frequenting places where the air was cooler and drier. Medieval doctors also suggested that people bathe less often, based on the idea that bathing opens the pores too much and thereby allows corrupted air to enter the body.

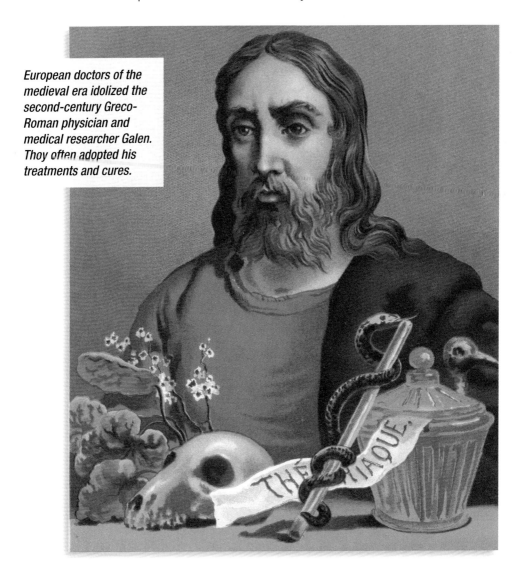

European doctors of the medieval era idolized the second-century Greco-Roman physician and medical researcher Galen. They often adopted his treatments and cures.

# Villages Beset by Wolves

In addition to the many people who died from the plague in Europe, numerous animals perished as well. Of the creatures that survived, some appeared to sense that human society was in a disordered state and began moving into abandoned and sparsely populated villages. In Germany in 1349, a local chronicler described a disturbing increase in the number of wolves threatening people. Those dangerous beasts, the account states, roamed around in packs at night and were sometimes seen during the daytime. In many villages, he said, the wolves

> did not slake their thirst for human blood by lurking in secret places . . . but boldly entered open houses and tore children from their mothers' sides. Indeed, they not only attacked children, but armed men, and overcame them. . . . They seemed no longer wild animals, but demons. Other creatures forsook [left behind] their woods. [For example,] ravens in innumerable flocks flew over the towns with loud croaking. The kite [a bird of prey] and the vulture were heard in the air, [and] on houses the cuckoos and owls alighted and filled the night with their mournful lament.

Quoted in Otto Friedrich, *The End of the World: A History.* New York: Fromm International, 1994, p. 125.

## A Wide Array of Futile Treatments

Such measures were useless, which contributed to large numbers of people contracting the plague. For those victims, doctors prescribed a fairly wide array of treatments, including an old standard—namely, getting plenty of bed rest and drinking a lot of fluids. This was sound advice as a general approach to healthy living, but by itself, it was not nearly enough to treat an illness as deadly as the Black Death.

Another futile treatment offered by physicians—bleeding—was equally ineffective against the plague. Indeed, it was also detrimental to the health of *any* sick person. This so-called treatment consisted of opening one or more of a patient's veins and then allowing "corrupted" blood to drain out into a bowl. Unfortunately for the patient, this procedure only succeeded in making him or her weaker. It was also common for doctors to try to help plague victims by opening and draining their buboes. Because they knew nothing about the existence of germs, they did not realize that large numbers of bacteria still remained inside the body, where they continued to multiply.

Still another prevalent anti-plague treatment was to apply certain substances directly to the intact buboes in hopes that this would make them recede. Such salves contained an exotic mix of ingredients, including shredded lily roots, tree resins, and human excrement. On doctors' orders, many other patients drank powdered gold or other granulated metals mixed with water. Because ingesting metals in such large doses is toxic, this so-called treatment ended up either making patients feel even worse or outright killing them before the plague did.

## Sanitation Rules and Quarantines

Despite these meager, useless attempts to save victims of the awful pandemic, there were notable exceptions to that rule. They consisted of the few doctors and other individuals who correctly suspected the disease might be somehow contagious. Their efforts, even if minor in the greater scheme of things, surely kept the disease from spreading as far as it might have in some regions and saved at least a few lives. One of these positive approaches to the plague's assault was to impose travel restrictions in some towns or districts. Another approach took the form of town councils enacting sanitation ordinances, or rules, in their areas. Moreover, some towns went a step further and introduced quarantines, in which plague victims were kept fully separate from healthy people.

In May 1348, for instance, officials in the Italian town of Pistoia issued a public decree that listed several anti-plague ordinances. "No citizen of Pistoia," the document stated, in part, "shall in any way dare or presume to go to [neighboring] Pisa or Lucca." Likewise, no person was allowed to travel from those towns to Pistoia. When people did make such trips, soldiers watching the roads stopped them and made them pay a fine of fifty lira, which was a hefty sum in that time and place. The travelers also had to turn back and return to their hometowns. Other rules imposed in the decree included the following:

No person [shall] dare or presume in any way to bring [to Pistoia] any used cloth, either linen or woolen, for use as clothing for men or women or for bedclothes on penalty of [paying] 200 lira. . . . The bodies of the dead [cannot be] removed from the place in which they are found unless first such a body has been placed in a wooden casket covered by a lid secured with nails, so that no stench can issue forth from it. . . . In order to avoid the foul stench which the bodies of the dead give off . . . any ditch in which a dead body is to be buried must be dug under ground to a depth of 2.5 braccia [or arm's length] by the measure of the city of Pistoia.[38]

## Major New Rules in Venice

Town officials in the famous northern Italian metropolis of Venice also issued comparable ordinances in 1348. One rule stated that any Venetian who had perished from the Black Death must be buried at a depth of at least 5 feet (1.5 m). In addition, infected persons who were still living had to be quarantined for forty days. This was accomplished by taking them to some nearby uninhabited islands. They were supplied with food, water, blankets, and other basic essentials needed to survive the forty-day stay. During that interval, no foreign vessels were allowed to dock either at the islands or in Venice itself. (The officials chose the number forty out of respect for God; forty days was the amount of time that Jesus fasted in the wilderness, as related in the Bible.)

These efforts to fight the plague were earnest and diligent. Yet over the course of the following eighteen months the disease killed at least one hundred thousand Venetians, about 60 percent of the city's population. The death lists included large numbers of physicians; worse, of the doctors who survived, a majority of them fled to parts unknown, leaving their patients to suffer and often die. A notable exception was a physician named Francesco. He remained at his post throughout the pandemic and when asked later why he did not abandon his countrymen, as his colleagues had, he replied, "I would rather die here than live elsewhere."[39]

Similar efforts to slow down the pandemic occurred all over Europe. Some regulations, such as those issued at Pistoia, were well-thought-out and wisely attempted to guard the local food supply. In this regard, butchers were especially singled out, based on the supposition that perhaps tainted meat was a cause of the plague. Thus, people who prepared and sold meat received long lists of detailed and exacting regulations. "Butchers and retailers of meat," the Pistoia authorities declared, "shall not stable horses or allow any mud or dung in the shop or other place where they sell meat, or in or near their storehouse, or on the roadway outside. Nor shall they slaughter animals in a stable or keep flayed [skinned] carcasses in a stable or in any other place where there is dung."[40]

## Forgiveness Through Self-Torture?

Although many Europeans saw the disease as a natural phenomenon, others viewed it as something less natural and more spiritual. It was a punishment sent by God, they insisted. Therefore, the only realistic way to stop it was to apologize to God and beg for forgiveness.

A great many of those Europeans who felt this way and acted on it came to be called flagellants, from the word *flagellate,* meaning "to punish by whipping." Romanian scholar Catalin Negru explains that they were "groups of people of both genders and of all ages that, as a sign of penitence, publicly whipped their bodies. These had the role of purifiers of the soul, who mistreat themselves without mercy in order to absolve the sins of themselves and of others."[41]

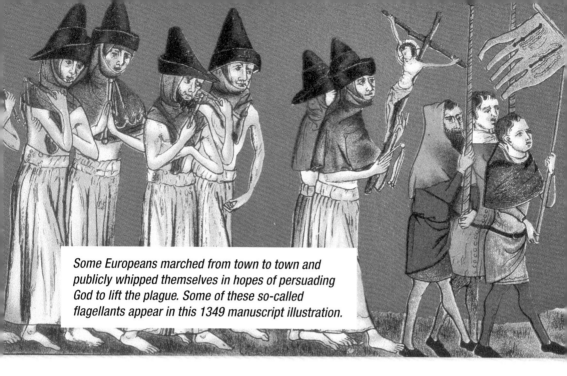

*Some Europeans marched from town to town and publicly whipped themselves in hopes of persuading God to lift the plague. Some of these so-called flagellants appear in this 1349 manuscript illustration.*

Numerous groups of these penitents formed across the continent during the plague's late 1340s onslaught. Numbering as few as a couple dozen and as many as a few thousand, flagellants wandered from town to town and sometimes country to country. Reaching a town's main square, where they could expect to attract the most attention, they stripped themselves to the waist and struck themselves with whips until they bled. There was no way to avoid the blood because the whips they employed, called scourges, were purposely designed to slash a person's flesh. One eyewitness of the era, German chronicler Heinrich of Herford, described a scourge as a wooden stick from which hung three strands, each bearing several knots. He continued,

> Through the knots were thrust iron spikes as sharp as needles, which penetrated about the length of a grain of wheat or a little more beyond the knots. With such scourges they beat themselves on their naked bodies so that they became swollen and blue, and blood ran down to the ground and spattered the walls of the churches in which they scourged themselves.[42]

These displays of self-torture were intended to re-create the beating that, according to the New Testament, Jesus received just before he was crucified. The flagellants hoped to show God that humans were genuinely sorry for their prior sins. But in order to do so, they reasoned, they first had to get his attention, and to accomplish that, simply whipping themselves might not be enough. Therefore, the beatings needed to be part of a larger-scale, more dramatic ceremony that included prayers, sermons, hymn singing, and more.

## Gone Like Ghosts in the Night

Thus, in each public ceremony, after the flagellants beat themselves for ten or fifteen minutes, they switched to an even more intense activity in which all but two of them lay face down on the ground. The two still standing, each of whom bore the title "master," strolled among the prostrate members. The masters used whips, and sometimes wooden sticks, to flog their comrades' backsides, which increased the outflow of blood. While administering this punishment, the masters called out to Jesus's mother, Mary. In her name, they said, the people on the ground should promise never to sin again, and the prostrate members made that promise aloud, perhaps repeating it many times.

> "Our journey's done in the holy name;/Jesus himself to Jerusalem came."[43]
>
> —From a hymn sung by the flagellants while flogging themselves

Next, at a master's signal, everyone knelt before a tall cross that signified the one on which Jesus met his end. For a while they listened to a sermon delivered by one of the masters. Following that, and maybe at other intervals during the ceremony, the flagellants marched in a circle while singing sad songs, among them one with the refrain, "Our journey's done in the holy name; / Jesus himself to Jerusalem came; / his cross he bore in his holy hand; / help us, savior of all the land.[43]

Some of the townspeople who witnessed these bizarre displays sympathized with the self-torturers and, at times, even

## Killing Some and Sparing Others

One of the most peculiar aspects of the Black Death was that some people who were exposed to it never caught it. Indeed, the disease appeared to kill some and spare others without any sort of discrimination. Although it sometimes wiped out entire families, some nearby neighbors who had had close contact with the victims somehow survived unscathed. Modern medical researchers say there are multiple reasons for this phenomenon. First, most often there was little or no direct person-to-person transmission of germs. Rather, the germs lived in the fleas, and if a victim no longer had any fleas in his or her house, a visitor was not likely to become exposed to the microbes. Much more dangerous was visiting a victim living in an area with poor sanitation. It tended to attract rats, which crawled with fleas, which in turn carried plague germs. Another factor was personal immunity. For various reasons, some people have stronger immune systems than others, so if the number of germs transmitted by a given flea was low, a person with strong immunity who was bitten by the insect had a good chance of surviving the disease.

joined in the activities. Others, however, felt that the flagellants were improperly performing a role that local priests normally did — interceding with God on humans' behalf. In fact, local clergymen increasingly saw the wandering penitents as a threat. In October 1349, therefore, Pope Clement issued a decree ordering all flagellants to be arrested. Under threat of imprisonment or even death, the flagellant groups disbanded during the three years that followed. This prompted a chronicler of that period to remark that they had vanished "as suddenly as they had come, like night phantoms or mocking ghosts."[44]

In a similar manner, by the middle of 1350, for reasons no one could explain, the plague itself had largely receded from Europe. Though this was good news, anyone who assumed that life would now go back to normal was fooling themselves. The truth was that, for better or worse, the continent and the lives of its residents had changed forever.

# CHAPTER FOUR

# Changes Wrought by the Plague

So catastrophic was the Black Death's visitation to Europe during the 1340s that nearly every aspect of life underwent major, permanent change. Religious belief and worship were deeply affected. So were everyday customs, literature, and the arts.

However, probably the largest transformation of all was a profound alteration at all levels of Europe's social and economic structure. The widespread destruction brought about by the plague resulted in profound changes in the trading of goods and services, the right to own the fruits of one's labor, the relationship between bosses and workers, the normal breakdown of occupations in society, and the long-accepted hold on power by super-wealthy landowners. These and other societal changes altered the way people of all social classes viewed their world. In fact, many historians think that the far-reaching changes wrought by the plague constituted one of the key factors in Western civilization's transition from the medieval to the modern era.

## Manorial Estates Under Stress

One of the most significant modifications the Black Death brought about was a massive, fatal blow to medieval Europe's entrenched manorial system. That socioeconomic arrangement had as its underlying basis a combined residence and financial hub called the manor. It consisted of an extensive piece of land dominated by a big home—the manor house. It also featured several barns, workrooms, cottages, and other outbuildings along with horses, cattle, pigs, and other animals owned by the lord of the manor.

In a way, the manor also included the peasants who raised the estate's animals and grew crops in its fields. Technically, those workers were not slaves because the lord did not own them outright. But they were, in both theory and reality, bound to remain the owner's servants for as long he liked, and that was most often for life. These so-called serfs owed the lord loyalty and had to give him a hefty portion of all crops they grew or products they manufactured on his property. Legally speaking, serfs *could* leave a manor and settle somewhere else. If they did so, however, they no longer had a ready source of food, nor did they enjoy the legal and military protection the lord had long provided them. Therefore, the vast majority of serfs stayed put, and the manorial system chugged along, affording rich landowners a built-in source of cheap labor.

The initial stress on the manorial system created by the bubonic plague was a rapid depletion of labor. The disease killed so many serfs that a large portion of European manors lost close to half, and sometimes up to three-quarters or more, of their workers. Guillaume de Machaut, a French poet who witnessed this devastation, remarked, "Many have certainly heard it commonly said how in [1349], out of one hundred [workers on a manor] there remained but nine. Thus it happened that for lack of people many a splendid farm was left untilled. No one plowed the fields, bound the cereals, and took in the grapes."[45]

## Crisis for Nobility, Power for Peasants

The landowning nobles experienced a crisis unlike any they had faced before. With far fewer tenant farmers and other workers

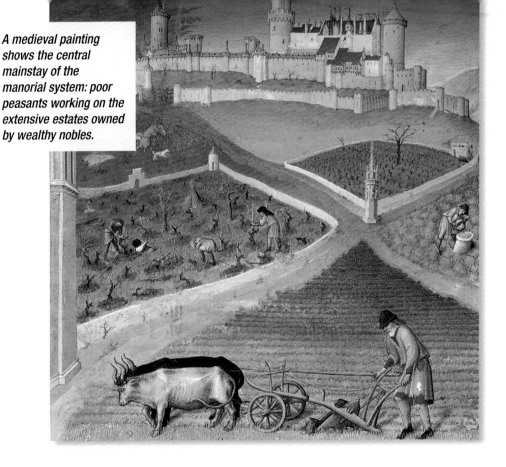

A medieval painting shows the central mainstay of the manorial system: poor peasants working on the extensive estates owned by wealthy nobles.

to run the big manors, they found it difficult to run their estates properly. Thus, they made far less profit than before.

Meanwhile, the surviving serfs dwelling on those estates suddenly realized that they now possessed considerable bargaining power. With local workforces depleted nearly everywhere, the landowners could not readily find replacements for peasants who threatened to leave. This meant that those lower-class workers could make certain demands on the manor lords. One such demand was the right to rent or lease the lands on which they lived, which gave them more say in how their parcels were managed.

At the same time, as scholar Robert S. Gottfried explains, depopulation and the scarcity of agricultural workers made the remaining workers far more valuable. As a result,

wages rose rapidly. [At] Cuxham Manor in England, a plowman who was paid 2 shillings a week in 1347 received 7 shillings in 1349, and 10 shillings [by] 1350. The result was a dramatic rise in standards of living for those in the lower [socioeconomic classes]. Day laborers not only received higher wages, but asked for and got lunches of meat pies and golden ale.[46]

For many wealthy landowners, the plague seemed to have turned their traditional world almost upside down. Traditional social roles and values frequently altered in ways that upper-class folk viewed as perplexing and disturbing. It seemed shocking to the nobility that the peasants had dared to take advantage of the changes caused by the plague's huge death toll. Furthermore, poorer folk, who did numerous types of jobs in the towns, also demanded and obtained higher wages. Thus, commoners were now able to enjoy a wide range of goods, services, and customs normally reserved for the wealthy elites. In 1363, Italian historian Matteo Villani commented that many common folk no longer recognized the superiority of the rich. Instead, the poor had the gall to demand "the dearest and most delicate foods for their sustenance; and they married at their will, while children and common women clad themselves in all the fair and costly garments of the [upper-class] ladies dead by [the plague]."[47]

> "Common women clad themselves in all the fair and costly garments of the [upper-class] ladies dead by [the plague]."[47]
>
> —Italian historian Matteo Villani

## Trying to Keep the Commoners in Check

As the disease raged across the continent, certain occupations became considerably more in demand than they had been before. Particularly sought-after were gravediggers, for example. This was not surprising considering the vast numbers of bodies that required burial. Also seen as high-value workers were doctors to help the sick and priests to administer last rites to the dead.

Aware of the increased need for their services, many of these individuals raised their fees. "Many chaplains and hired parish priests would not serve without excessive pay," an Englishman of that time wrote. On occasion, he added, this practice sparked outrage. An angry bishop in the town of Rochester "commanded these [priests] to serve at the same salaries [as before], under pain of suspension."[48]

A similar situation existed with the prices of goods. So many skilled artisans and craftspeople died during the pandemic, for instance, that far fewer goods were created. This included clothing, fabrics, pottery, building materials, and luxury goods. Not surprisingly, this made the items that *were* manufactured more valuable and thereby more expensive on the open market.

Big landowners and other wealthy people were able to pay the higher prices. So were some of the members of the lower classes, thanks to their new higher earnings. According to Villani, formerly poor people who were not used to extravagance sometimes indulged in various luxuries, including eating more meat and wearing stylish clothes.

Many well-to-do and noble individuals were disgruntled that people they had long viewed as inferiors were enjoying both social clout and comforts usually reserved for the wealthy class. Most high-placed persons of that era tended to see this as unnatural and a threat to the traditional social order. The nobles and other rich folk who controlled town and national governments across Europe tried to prevent such changes from taking place by passing new laws. Sumptuary laws, as they were known, placed limits on displays of luxury and extravagance by members of the lower classes. A few of these laws passed during the plague years, but most were enacted in the plague's aftermath, in the decades following 1350.

Sumptuary laws designed to keep the commoners in check were passed in England not long after the plague receded. These laws varied depending on family income. Under one such law, women from modest-income families could wear moderately

# The Peasants Demand Their Fair Share

As a result of the changes caused by the Black Death, members of the lower classes boldly began to demand more rights and better treatment. Upper-class individuals tended to resent this new behavior by people they considered their inferiors. In 1363, Italian chronicler Matteo Villani listed some lower-class demands for better wages and benefits: "Serving girls and unskilled women with no experience in service and stable boys want at least 12 florins per year, and the most arrogant among them 18 or 24 florins per year, and so also nurses and minor artisans working with their hands want three times [the] usual pay."

Many miles to the north of Italy, in plague-ravaged England, a similar situation was unfolding. Upset over the demands being made by local peasants, an English country gentleman named John Gower complained in 1375, "[A] shepherd and cowherd demand more for their labor than the master-baliff [farm manager]. . . . Labor is now at so high a price that he who will order his business aright must pay five or six shillings now for what [used to] cost him two. Poor and small folk demand to be better fed than their masters."

Quoted in David Herlihy, *The Black Death and the Transformation of the West.* Cambridge, MA: Harvard University Press, 1997, pp. 48–49.

Quoted in Otto Friedrich, *The End of the World: A History.* New York: Fromm International, 1994, p. 135.

priced furs but could *not* wear the white fur of an ermine, which was reserved for the rich. Those same women could wear jewelry, but only in their hair. Meanwhile, the very poorest women were prohibited from wearing any jewelry, and their clothing had to be made from plain, inexpensive cloth.

Members of the aristocratic classes throughout Europe hoped that these laws would restrain members of the lower classes and, over time, reinforce the boundaries between them. The ultimate outcome was very different, however. As has been the case with a majority of sumptuary laws installed in various places and historical periods, they largely failed. In post-plague fourteenth-century Europe, so many commoners gained higher living standards and increased economic clout that they became a social force that could no longer be held back.

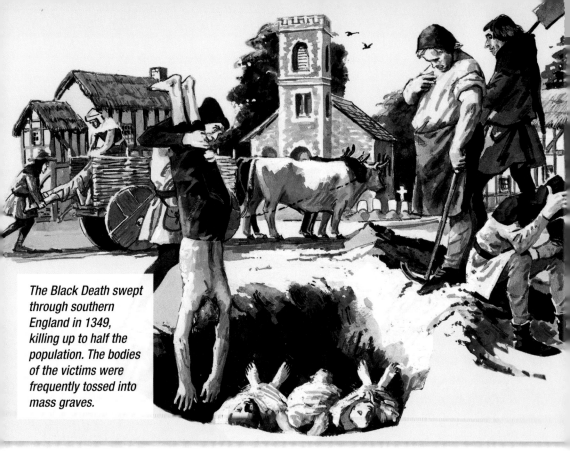

The Black Death swept through southern England in 1349, killing up to half the population. The bodies of the victims were frequently tossed into mass graves.

## Worry Leads to Restrictive New Laws

The societal elites who passed the sumptuary laws, both during and after the plague's onslaught, became desperate when they saw that the laws failed to have the desired effect. Fearing that society's traditional power structure might crumble, a number of local and national officials and rulers resorted to more forceful means to maintain their control over the lower classes. One frequent approach was to pass laws that prohibited serfs from leaving the manors where they had spent most of their lives. Other laws sought to stop commoners from switching jobs to obtain higher pay and improved social positions. Still other laws created maximum amounts that any lower-class individual could earn in a specific occupation. The intent of these laws, scholar Philip Ziegler points out, was to force a return to the wages and prices of the preplague era. Government leaders, he says, realized that this could never be achieved as long as laborers were free to move from one employer to another in search of higher wages and so long as employers were free to woo away laborers from their neighbors with [tempting] offers. By restricting the right of an employee to leave his place of work . . . they hoped to re-create the conditions that pertained before the plague and maintain them forever.[49]

Some people paid no heed to these laws and, as a result, were either forced to pay large fines or were arrested and prosecuted. That helped to make these statutes extremely unpopular among all but the wealthiest families. The situation in England was a case in point. An English chronicler of that era, Henry Knighton, stated in his account of the plague years and their immediate aftermath that the commoners refused to observe the new and restrictive rules the government had imposed. Thus, government officials levied heavy fines on them. Afterward, Knighton continues, "the king had many laborers arrested, and sent them to prison; many withdrew themselves and went into the forests and woods; and those who were [caught] were heavily fined. Their ringleaders were made to swear that they would not take daily wages beyond the ancient custom, and then were freed from prison."[50]

> "The king had many laborers arrested, and sent them to prison; many withdrew themselves and went into the forests and woods; and those who were [caught] were heavily fined."[50]
>
> —English chronicler Henry Knighton

## Local Rebellions Erupt

This growing tendency to use strong-arm tactics to try to bring back the traditional social order only ended up further upsetting and angering the members of the lower classes. A growing number reacted by organizing into armed bands and staging rebellions of varying size. One of the largest of these uprisings took place in France in 1358. It gained the name "Jacquerie" based on the fact that French peasants were regularly referred to as "Jacques." The fourteenth-century French historian Jean Froissart described it, saying, in part, that a big mob of Jacques "gathered together without any other counsel [plan], and without any armor [wielding only] staves and knives, and so went to the house of a knight dwelling thereby, and broke up his house and slew the knight and the lady and all his children great and small and burned his house."[51]

Much larger was a 1381 revolt of former serfs that took place in southern England. Peasants numbering forty thousand or more marched on London, where the mob's leaders hoped to get an audience with King Richard II. According to Knighton, some mem-

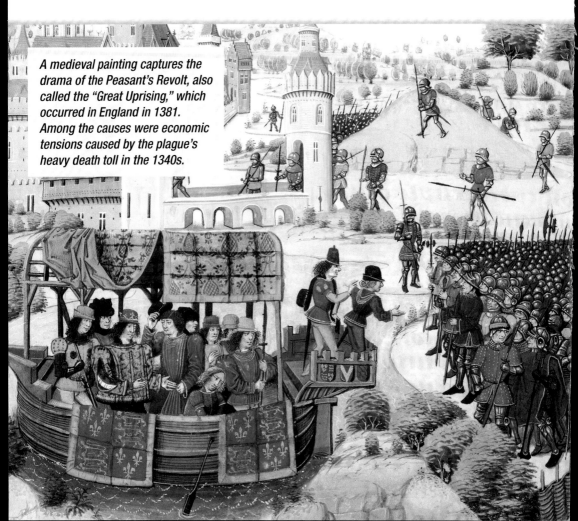

*A medieval painting captures the drama of the Peasant's Revolt, also called the "Great Uprising," which occurred in England in 1381. Among the causes were economic tensions caused by the plague's heavy death toll in the 1340s.*

bers of the crowd reached the Tower of London, where a large group of knights and soldiers encircled the king in an attempt to protect him. The peasant leaders sent word that they did not seek to overthrow Richard; rather, they merely wanted to present him with their grievances. Hearing this, the king bravely left his soldiers behind and, accompanied by only two or three guards, faced the horde of protesters outside the city's defensive walls. According to an English chronicler of that period, a rebel leader then stepped forward and respectfully but firmly told the monarch

> that they had been seriously oppressed by many hardships and that their condition of servitude was unbearable, and that they neither could nor would endure it longer. The king, for the sake of peace, and on account of the violence of the times, and yielding to their petition, granted them a charter with the great seal, to the effect that all men in the kingdom of England should be free and of free condition.[52]

Unfortunately for the peasants, that specific agreement turned out to be meaningless; later that year, under heavy pressure from his chief nobles, Richard canceled it. Nevertheless, England's lower classes did make major gains during further negotiations with the monarchy. During the decade that followed, the government agreed to reduce a tax it had earlier imposed on all commoners and that was widely seen as unfair and burdensome. The government also agreed to allow most peasant farmers and laborers to work wherever they wanted. In times past, the manorial system had made it exceedingly difficult for most peasants to leave their lord's estate.

## A Pioneering Path to the Future

Historians have noted many other socioeconomic effects of the plague's fourteenth-century assault on Europe. Among them was a marked reduction in the number of wealthy landowners on much of the continent. Their numbers fell as their estates

## French Peasants on a Killing Spree

In 1358 French peasants rebelled over restrictions placed on them by the upper classes. During the rebellion, the peasants attacked several manor houses and killed their well-to-do inhabitants, as reported by fourteenth-century French historian Jean Froissart:

> [The marauders] went to another castle, and took the knight thereof and bound him fast to a stake, and then violated his wife and his daughter before his face and then slew the lady and his daughter and all his other children, and then slew the knight by great torment and burned and beat down the castle. And so they did to diverse other castles and good houses; and they multiplied so that they were six thousand, and ever as they went forward they increased [in number], so that every gentleman fled from them and took their wives and children with them . . . and left their house void and their goods therein. These mischievous people thus assembled without captain . . . robbed, burned, and slew all gentlemen that they could lay hands on, [and] did such shameful deeds that no human creature ought to think on any such, and he that did most mischief was most praised [by the others]. I dare not write the horrible deeds that they did.

Quoted in Internet Medieval Source Book, "Jean Froissart: On the Jacquerie, 1358," Fordham University, January 2, 2020. https://sourcebooks.fordham.edu.

lost value. The plague had wiped out so many of the serfs who labored on those estates that many of the owners could no longer turn a profit. In the words of German historian Friedrich Lütge, when the Black Death largely receded during the early 1350s, huge numbers of land plots once occupied by peasants lay abandoned. That severely reduced the incomes of the big landowners, some of whom had to sell their estates to keep from going bankrupt.

Meanwhile, Lütge writes, on those few estates that still used serfs, those laborers were far more valued than before simply because they were fewer in number and harder to find. Such a worker was now "able to lessen his obligations [to the manor lord] in many ways because he was in high demand. There was, moreover, a decline in the purchasing power of money. . . . Thus, [some of] the landlords became impoverished [and] the German knightly order was reduced to bankruptcy."[53]

Driven by the momentous changes resulting from the chaos and tragedy of the Black Death, the manorial system had largely vanished from most of Europe by the mid-1400s. The socioeconomic class structure on which European life had been built saw the start of a dramatic transformation. The nobles had lost much power and influence, whereas the lower classes had gained both economic clout and the opportunity for further advancement. In the fullness of time, these trends were destined to lead Europeans down a pioneering path to a new society—the one today referred to as "modern." As David Herlihy puts it, "Out of the havoc of plague, Europe adopted what can well be called the modern Western mode of [thought and] behavior."[54]

# SOURCE NOTES

### Introduction: A Crucial Turning Point in History

1. Quoted in Rosemary Horrox, trans. and ed., *The Black Death.* Manchester, UK: Manchester University Press, 1994, pp. 19–20.
2. Giovanni Boccaccio, *Decameron,* trans. Mark Musa and Peter Bondanella. New York: W.W. Norton, 1982, pp. 10–11.
3. Philip Ziegler, *The Black Death.* New York: Harper and Row, 2009, p. 279.
4. Richard Conniff, "How Pandemics Have Changed Us," *National Geographic,* August 2020, p. 73.

### Chapter One: The Black Death Assaults Europe

5. Horrox, *The Black Death,* p. 3.
6. William H. McNeill, *Plagues and Peoples.* New York: Random House, 1998, p. 176.
7. Quoted in Horrox, *The Black Death,* p. 17.
8. Quoted in Martha Carlin, "The Black Death in the British Isles," Department of History, University of Wisconsin–Milwaukee. https://sites.uwm.edu/carlin.
9. Quoted in David Herlihy, *The Black Death and the Transformation of the West.* Cambridge, MA: Harvard University Press, 1997, p. 24.
10. Quoted in Decameron Web, "Marchionne di Coppo di Stefano Buonaiuti," Italian Studies Department, Brown University, February 18, 2010. www.brown.edu.
11. Quoted in Horrox, *Black Death,* pp. 55–56.
12. Quoted in Carlin, "The Black Death in the British Isles."
13. Quoted in Decameron Web, "Marchionne di Coppo di Stefano Buonaiuti."
14. Herlihy, *The Black Death and the Transformation of the West,* p. 25.

15. Giovanni Boccaccio, *Decameron,* trans. G.H. McWilliams. London: Penguin, 1972, pp. 7–8.
16. Quoted in Horrox, *The Black Death,* pp. 31–32.
17. Quoted in Horrox, *The Black Death,* p. 17.

## Chapter Two: Trying to Explain the Unexplainable
18. Jean de Venette, *The Chronicle of Jean de Venette,* trans. Jean Birdsall, ed. Richard A. Newhall. New York: Columbia University Press, 1953, pp. 48–49.
19. De Venette, *The Chronicle of Jean de Venette,* p. 49.
20. Quoted in Horrox, *The Black Death,* pp. 160–61.
21. Horrox, *The Black Death,* pp. 100–101.
22. James C. Giblin, *When Plague Strikes: The Black Death, Smallpox, AIDS.* New York: HarperCollins, 1997, pp. 32–33.
23. Shaina Lucas, "The Unfortunate Scapegoats of the Black Death Were Mainly Heretics, Jews, and Witches," History Collection. https://historycollection.com.
24. Quoted in Horrox, *The Black Death,* p. 45.
25. Quoted in Horrox, *The Black Death,* p. 208.
26. Quoted in Internet History Sourcebooks Project, "Jewish History Sourcebook: The Black Death and the Jews 1348–1349 CE," Fordham University, January 2, 2020. https://source books.fordham.edu.
27. Quoted in Horrox, *The Black Death,* pp. 113–14.
28. Quoted in Mary A. Devlin, ed., *The Sermons of Thomas Brinton.* Vol. 1. London: Royal Historical Society, 1954, p. 38.
29. Quoted in Horrox, *The Black Death,* p. 126.
30. Boccaccio, *Decameron,* trans. Musa and Bondanella, p. 6.
31. Barbara W. Tuchman, *A Distant Mirror: The Calamitous 14th Century.* New York: Ballantine, 1996, p. 109.
32. Quoted in Internet History Sourcebooks Project, "Boccaccio: *The Decameron,* 'Introduction,'" Fordham University, January 2, 2020. https://sourcebooks.fordham.edu.
33. Quoted in Horrox, *The Black Death,* p. 36.
34. Quoted in Horrox, *The Black Death,* p. 36.
35. Quoted in Herlihy, *The Black Death and the Transformation of the West,* p. 63.

## Chapter Three: Attempts to Deal with the Plague
36. Quoted in Phoebe Roma Lauren, "Primary Sources," Black Death. https://phoeberomalaurentheblackdeath2.weebly.com.

37. Quoted in Lauren, "Primary Sources."
38. Quoted in Plague and Public Health in Renaissance Europe, "Pistoia: Ordinances for Sanitation in a Time of Mortality," Institute for Advanced Technology in the Humanities, University of Virginia, October 28, 1994. www2.iath.virginia.edu.
39. Quoted in Ziegler, *The Black Death,* p. 38.
40. Quoted in Horrox, *The Black Death,* pp. 198–99.
41. Catalin Negru, "*History of the Apocalypse:* The Black Plague and the Flagellants," Reason and Religion, 2020. https://reasonandreligion.org.
42. Quoted in Ziegler, *The Black Death,* p. 67.
43. Quoted in Otto Friedrich, *The End of the World: A History.* New York: Fromm International, 1994, p. 126.
44. Quoted in Friedrich, *The End of the World,* p. 129.

## Chapter Four: Changes Wrought by the Plague
45. Quoted in Herlihy, *The Black Death and the Transformation of the West,* p. 41.
46. Robort S. Gottfried, *The Black Death: Natural and Human Disaster in Medieval Europe.* New York: Macmillan, 1985, p. 94.
47. Quoted in Alison Futrell, "Plague Readings," History of Western Civilization: From the Rise of Cities to the Counter-Reformation (TRAD 102), University of Arizona. www.u.arizona.edu.
48. Quoted in Futrell, "Plague Readings."
49. Ziegler, *The Black Death,* p. 199.
50. Quoted in Leon Bernard and Theodore B. Hodges, eds., *Readings in European History.* New York: Macmillan, 1958, p. 213.
51. Quoted in Internet Medieval Source Book, "Jean Froissart: On the Jacquerie, 1358," Fordham University, January 2, 2020. https://sourcebooks.fordham.edu.
52. Quoted in Bernard and Hodges, *Readings in European History,* p. 215.
53. Friedrich Lütge, "Germany: The Black Death and a Structural Revolution in Socioeconomic History," in *The Black Death: A Turning Point in History?,* ed. William M. Bowsky. New York: Holt, Rinehart and Winston, 1978, p. 84.
54. Herlihy, *The Black Death and the Transformation of the West,* p. 57.

# FOR FURTHER RESEARCH

## Books

Barbara Krasner, *Bubonic Plague: How the Black Death Changed the World.* North Mankato, MN: Raintree, 2019.

Emily J. Mahoney, *The Black Death: Bubonic Plague Attacks Europe.* New York: Lucent Press, 2017.

Don Nardo, *COVID-19 and Other Pandemics: A Comparison.* San Diego: ReferencePoint, 2021.

Stephen Porter, *Black Death.* Gloucestershire, UK: Amberley, 2018.

## Internet Sources

BBC History Extra, "Black Death Facts: Your Guide to 'The Worst Catastrophe in Recorded History,'" May 12, 2020. www.historyextra.com.

Winston Black, "What Was the Black Death?," Live Science, December 12, 2019. www.livescience.com.

Mark Cartwright, "Black Death," Ancient History Encyclopedia, March 28, 2020. www.ancient.eu.

Centers for Disease Control and Prevention, "Plague," November 26, 2019. www.cdc.gov.

Jenny Howard, "Plague Was One of History's Deadliest Diseases—Then We Found a Cure," *National Geographic*, July 6, 2020. www.nationalgeographic.com.

Emily Kasriel, "What Plague Art Tells Us About Today," BBC Culture, May 18, 2020. www.bbc.com.

Nicholas LePan, "Visualizing the History of Pandemics," Visual Capitalist, March 14, 2020. www.visualcapitalist.com.

Science Museum, "Bubonic Plague: The First Pandemic," April 25, 2019. www.sciencemuseum.org.uk.

Lizzie Wade, "From Black Death to Fatal Flu, Past Pandemics Show Why People on the Margins Suffer Most," *Science*, May 14, 2020. www.sciencemag.org.

World Health Organization, "Plague." 2019. www.who.int.

# INDEX

# PICTURE CREDITS

# Important Events During the Black Death

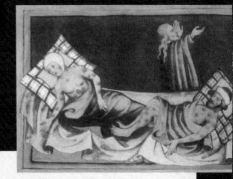

## ca. 1331
An outbreak of bubonic plague occurs in southwestern China and soon spreads to Mongolia and other parts of Asia.

## October 1347
Another ship from Kaffa reaches Sicily, where the disease kills half the population.

## May 1347
The siege of Kaffa ends and European sailors carry the plague to Constantinople, located on the Black Sea's southern rim.

1330   /   1345      1346      1347

## November 1347
The Black Death reaches France and swiftly spreads through the countryside.

## 1345
The Mongols, some of them infected with plague, lay siege to Kaffa, on the Crimean peninsula, and spread the disease to the town.

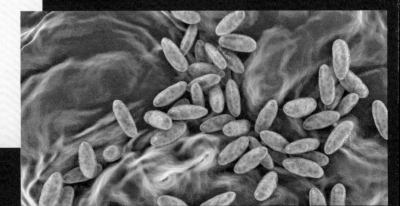

# CONTENTS

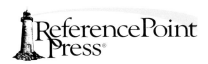

About the Author

Classical historian and award-winning author Don Nardo has written numerous volumes about historical, scientific, and medical topics, including *Migrant Mother* (nominated for eight best book of the year awards), *Tycho Brahe* (winner of the National Science Teaching Association's best book of the year), *Deadliest Dinosaurs*, *The History of Pandemics*, and *The History of Science*. Nardo, who also composes and arranges orchestral music, lives with his wife, Christine, in Massachusetts.

© 2022 ReferencePoint Press, Inc.
Printed in the United States

**For more information, contact:**
ReferencePoint Press, Inc.
PO Box 27779
San Diego, CA 92198
www.ReferencePointPress.com

LIBRARY OF CONGRESS CATALOGING-IN-PUBLICATION DATA

Names: Nardo, Don, 1947- author.
Title: Bubonic plague and the Black Death / by Don Nardo.
Description: San Diego, CA : ReferencePoint Press, Inc., 2022. | Series: Historic pandemics and plagues | Includes bibliographical references and index.
Identifiers: LCCN 2020056773 (print) | LCCN 2020056774 (ebook) | ISBN 9781678200985 (library binding) | ISBN 9781678200992 (ebook)
Subjects: LCSH: Black Death--Europe--History--Juvenile literature. | Plague--Europe--History--Juvenile literature.
Classification: LCC RC178.A1 N38 2022  (print) | LCC RC178.A1  (ebook) | DDC 614.5/732--dc23
LC record available at https://lccn.loc.gov/2020056773
LC ebook record available at https://lccn.loc.gov/2020056774

# Bubonic Plague and the Black Death

Don Nardo

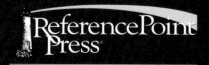

San Diego, CA